I dedicate this book to the medical professionals, caretakers, and friends who continue to support my recovery journey. They are true superheroes. Their patience, understanding, and straight talk have enabled me to develop a successful recovery strategy. Yes, it is a long and hard journey but their encouragement has given me the strength to not give up.

CONTENTS

Rebound - Thriving After Stroke: Encouragement and Tips for Men and Their Caregivers

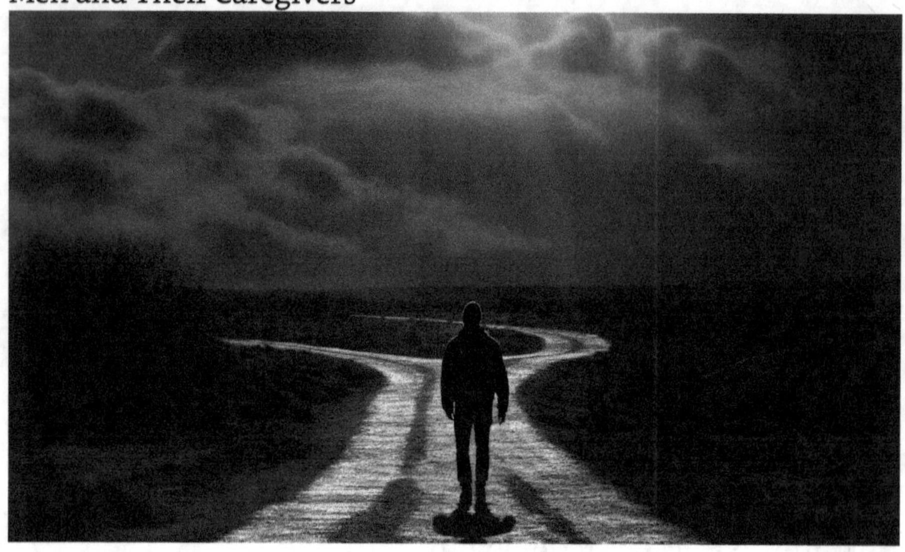

Written by Marc E. Parham (www.marcparham.com)

ISBN: 9798856223032

WHY I WROTE
THIS BOOK

I had a stroke in 2020 during the Covid crisis. As you will read, this stoke changed my entire way of life. During my recovery, my cardiologist recognized that I was an author and suggested that I write a book about my recovery journey focused on what men have to contend with.

She asked me to write this book because many men have had strokes that could have been avoided had they followed the instructions and medications recommended by their physicians.

Through my discussions with men recovering from stroke and her experiences, we discussed the primary impacting factor: most men did not follow their physician's instructions because the medications caused most men to deal with erectile dysfunction. Many men made other changes in their lives that they assumed would help deal with their high blood pressure and diabetes issues so they would not have to take the medication causing the ED issues.

My cardiologist told me, "I can help correct the ED issue with medications and other treatments. This is much easier than replacing your heart". She only had to tell me this once.

I immediately started following the exact recommendations that my doctors prescribed.

I started charting my progress, which helped my doctors and I ensure my treatment that plan was working.

The other critical aspect of my recovery was working with my caregiver, a very close friend that I thank this day for allowing me to recover in her home, which I am sure was not easy dealing with an alpha male who was now dependent on others to assist him with regular daily activities.

Please read this book to help you on your recovery journey.

INTRODUCTION

My Story - *I am an African-American male. I was 59 years old and in good shape. Every weekend, I was either hiking, cycling, or running. I have worked out with a trainer for the last six years. I have been working in my own business, doing work I enjoy. I had been living on a boat at a marina for the past few years. I was a musician playing congas out with different bands. I have been able to travel internationally multiple times a year for the past few years. I was living what I thought was my best life.*

September 13, 2020, that all changed.

I had a devastating stroke; the left side of my body, among other things, just shut down. Just like that!

More detail to follow...

— Marc Parham

Rebound - Thriving After Stroke: Encouragement and Tips for Men and Their Caregivers is an essential resource for stroke patients and their caregivers. It is a comprehensive guide that offers practical advice, encouragement, and hope to those who have suffered a stroke.

Stroke is a leading cause of death and disability worldwide. It affects millions of people, and the impact can be devastating. Stroke can cause physical, cognitive, and emotional impairments that significantly affect a person's quality of life. While stroke recovery is a long and challenging journey, it is possible to regain independence and live a fulfilling life.

This book is essential because it provides stroke patients and their caregivers with valuable information and tools to help them navigate recovery. It offers practical advice on managing various aspects of stroke recovery, including mobility issues, cognitive impairments, emotional distress, fatigue, and weakness.

The book also guides how to deal with occupational limitations and offers tips on adapting to new roles and responsibilities. It addresses stroke patients' challenges in returning to work and provides strategies for overcoming these obstacles.

One of the unique aspects of this book is that it is specifically tailored to men who have suffered a stroke. It recognizes that men may face different challenges in their recovery journey and offers advice and encouragement relevant to their needs.

The book also acknowledges the critical role that caregivers play in stroke recovery. It provides tips on how caregivers can support their loved ones and care for themselves during this challenging time.

In conclusion, Thriving After Stroke: Encouragement and Tips for Men and Their Caregivers is an essential resource for stroke patients and their caregivers. It offers practical advice, encouragement, and hope to those who have suffered a stroke and provides a roadmap for navigating the recovery process. This book is a must-read for anyone who wants to thrive after a stroke.

THE PURPOSE OF THE BOOK

The purpose of this book is to provide encouragement and tips for men who have suffered from a stroke, as well as their caregivers. Stroke recovery can be challenging, but with the right mindset and tools, it is possible to thrive after a stroke.

This book is specifically tailored to men who have had a stroke, as they often face unique challenges during recovery. Men may struggle with mobility, cognitive impairments, emotional distress, fatigue and weakness, and occupational limitations. The information and advice provided in this book will help men navigate these challenges and achieve the best possible recovery.

One of the key themes of this book is the importance of mindset and attitude in stroke recovery.

Another important aspect of stroke recovery is physical rehabilitation. This book will provide an overview of the different types of rehabilitation available, including physical therapy, occupational therapy, and speech therapy. It will also offer tips for maximizing the benefits of rehabilitation, including setting goals and tracking progress.

For men struggling with emotional distress, the book will guide how to cope with depression, anxiety, and other mental health issues. It also advises communicating with loved ones and healthcare professionals about emotional needs.

The book will also address practical concerns, such as managing fatigue and weakness, adapting to occupational limitations, and navigating the healthcare system. It will provide tips for self-care, including exercise, nutrition, and stress management.

Overall, this book aims to provide men who have had a stroke and their caregivers with the support and guidance they need to thrive during the recovery process. With the right mindset, tools, and resources, achieving a fulfilling and meaningful life after a stroke is possible.

HOW STROKES AFFECT MEN DIFFERENTLY

My Story - *I woke up one day and fell over because the left side of my body was not working. As time passed, things started returning, so instead of rushing to the hospital, I held out, hoping things would continue improving. The next day, things did improve physically but were starting to change with my speech and mental capacity. People started saying I sounded funny. I spoke with a very close friend who knew the signs of stroke and they called the fire department for a health check on me. There begins my stroke recovery journey. A journey I am still on to this day. There are so many up-and-down days. Days living in fear of simple things like falling. My emotions are all over the place. I can be mean and hard to deal with, and my self-worth is always questioned. Not by those around me, but by me. How can I go from being a true alpha male to needing someone to walk with me so I can pace my steps and not fall. By the way, the falling thing? Get over it. It will happen. The funny thing, it is not a typical fall. You feel like it takes over five minutes to hit the ground.*

- Marc Parham

Strokes are one of the leading causes of death and disability worldwide, and they affect men and women differently. Men are more likely to suffer from strokes than women and are at a higher risk of experiencing severe symptoms and complications. We will explore how strokes affect men differently and provide tips and encouragement for stroke recovery for men and their caregivers.

The Warning Signs Men Ignore

Ok, men, things may not work just right as we age. When we visit the doctor, we know we will hear the whole watch out for your blood pressure and diabetes talk. Some of us are active and in decent shape. Some, like me, even became vegan and had a healthy diet. We may even experience a cardiac event. Ninty-nine percent of the men I have surveyed after a stroke said ED was one of the main reasons they were not taking the recommended blood pressure medication. My cardiologist told me she can fix erectile dysfunction easier than repairing your heart.

But then stroke happens!

The Relationship With Your Doctor

This won't take long. What relationship? A genuine relationship requires complete honesty. Have we been completely honest with our doctors? We are convinced that it is their job to find something wrong. We may even make them work to find it. Full disclosure is a must. How can doctors prescribe the correct medications if they don't know everything?

The Medications

Please take the time to research your prescribed medications—especially the side effects. You must know how they will affect you, especially when taken with other meds. You may also find other medications that work better. Discuss with your doctor. Your recovery is a joint effort. Your doctor will appreciate it.

Track Your Progress

You have to keep track of your numbers. Otherwise, the only numbers the doctor can use are the ones they measure when you go to appointments; we know how those will be.

Many phone applications will help you keep track of your vitals. They will connect via Bluetooth directly to your phone. This way, you can send the reports to your doctor to discuss your recovery progress.

The more your doctor knows, the better your treatment plan.

Listening To the Women in Our Lives

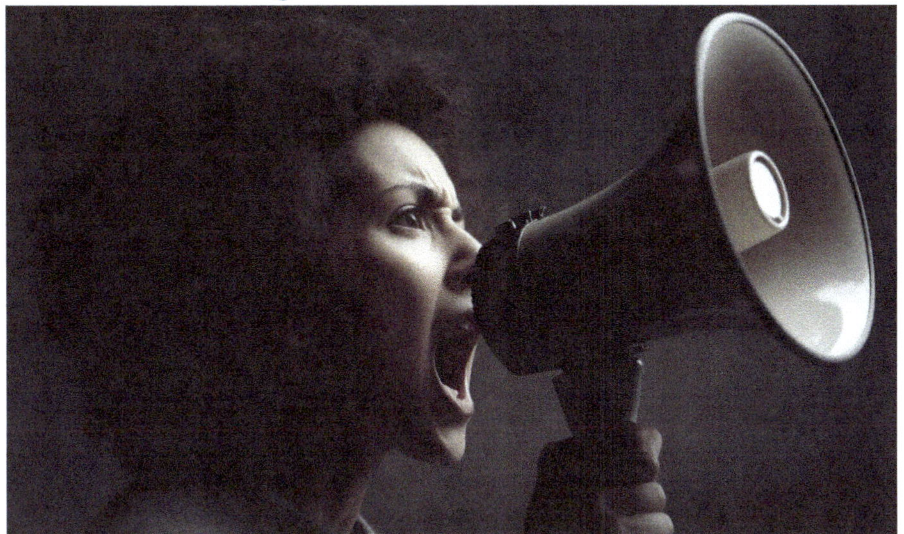

Yes, I said it! Women are very well versed in the whole dealing with medical doctors thing. They are taught very young about the importance of a relationship with a doctor. Women will tell us to get checked out over and over. We will eventually give in and are not surprised when the doctor finds something like we knew they would.

STROKE RECOVERY FOR MEN

My Story - *My first physical therapist asked me, "Do you want to walk out of here?" I said, "Yes." He said, "You must do everything we say even when we are not here to say it." That is what I did, even on the weekends when they were not there. I did walk out, although I was walking like Frankenstein. This recovery thing is a beast. Things you can do today you may not be able to do tomorrow. I need my cane one day; I feel like I can run a 5K the next day. It makes no sense. I need someone to help guide me. They may not know it, but I use them to pace my walking and sometimes as a buffer around other people so they don't do that head tilt thing and ask, "How are you doing?" or "Tell me what happened." Those two questions are the hardest to answer. Do I tell them how I am doing because I will feel differently fifteen minutes from now? Do I tell them what happened and go into PTSD, remembering the struggle, pain, and depression of my continued recovery? As I have said before, my emotions are all over the place. There are certain times I want to cry. As a man who has prided himself on his strength, you ask yourself, "Who wants a weak man?" This has been a very humbling experience. The only way I survive daily is to trust in God's process.*

- Marc Parham

Stroke recovery is a long and challenging process, and it can be especially difficult for men who may feel pressure to be strong and independent. Men may also be more hesitant to ask for help or show vulnerability, hindering their recovery. However, men must understand that stroke recovery is a team effort and must rely on their caregivers, healthcare providers, and support systems to achieve their goals.

Stroke Recovery for Men with Mobility Issues

Mobility issues are a common side effect of strokes, and they can significantly impact men's daily lives. Men may struggle with walking, balance, and coordination, making it difficult to perform simple tasks like getting dressed or going to the bathroom. Physical therapy and exercise can help improve mobility and prevent further complications, and caregivers can provide support and assistance as needed. No one wants to walk with a cane, but a cane may be necessary for a while. It will help to keep you from doing that falling thing, which is not very cool.

Stroke Recovery for Men with Cognitive Impairments

Cognitive impairments can also be a side effect of strokes, affecting men's ability to think clearly, remember things, and communicate effectively. Men may struggle with problem-solving, decision-making, and processing information, making participating in daily activities and social interactions difficult. Speech therapy, cognitive therapy, and memory aids can help improve cognitive function, and caregivers can provide emotional support and encouragement.

Stroke Recovery for Men with Emotional Distress

Emotional distress is common among stroke survivors, and men may experience feelings of depression, anxiety, and frustration.

Men may also feel a sense of loss of identity or purpose, especially if they were previously independent or active. Men must seek support from their healthcare providers, support groups, and loved ones and prioritize self-care activities that promote mental health and well-being.

Stroke Recovery for Men with Fatigue and Weakness

Fatigue and weakness are common side effects of strokes, and they can make it difficult for men to perform daily tasks and participate in activities they enjoy. Men may also experience muscle weakness or paralysis, limiting their mobility and independence. Exercise, physical, and occupational therapy can help improve strength and energy levels, and caregivers can provide support and assistance as needed.

Stroke Recovery for Men with Occupational Limitations

Occupational limitations are common among stroke survivors, and men may struggle to return to work or participate in activities that require physical or cognitive abilities. Men may also experience financial hardship or a sense of loss of purpose or identity due to their limitations.

Vocational rehabilitation, occupational therapy, and counseling can help men identify new career paths or hobbies that align with their abilities and interests.

Stroke patients with occupational limitations may experience difficulty with their work or daily routine. This can include difficulty with communication, memory, or physical tasks. Stroke patients need to work with their healthcare team and caregivers to develop a plan for returning to work or finding alternative ways to stay active and engaged.

In conclusion, strokes affect men differently, and stroke recovery requires a team effort and a holistic approach that addresses physical, cognitive, emotional, and occupational needs. Men and their caregivers should seek support from healthcare providers, support groups, and loved ones and prioritize self-care activities that promote mental and physical well-being. With perseverance and support, men can thrive after a stroke and regain their independence and quality of life.

THE STAGES OF STROKE RECOVERY

***My Story** - This is where the real journey begins. A journey that is yours alone. Many others have experienced stroke, but no stroke journey is like another. They may be similar, but not the same. It was the pain, daily brain fog, and learning to walk again. Combined with my stroke during Covid, I had to endure it alone with the hospital staff for about 30 days. My love goes out to the unsung superheroes, the nursing and rehabilitation staff. They kept it straight with me that if I wanted out with the possibility of living a near everyday life, I needed to do everything, I mean everything that they said, and to continue to do everything once I left the hospital. This is what I contribute to my recovery. The hardest part of recovery? What I can do today, I may not be able to do tomorrow, and this is after three years. This is also frustrating for me, and I am sure for those around me.*

- Marc Parham

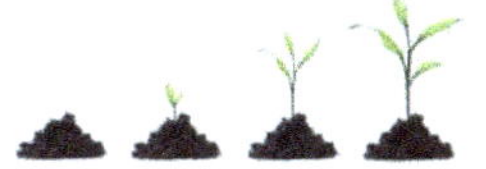

The stages of stroke recovery can vary from person to person, depending on the severity of the stroke and the individual's overall health. However, there are three primary stages of stroke recovery: acute, subacute, and chronic.

Acute Stage

The acute stage of stroke recovery typically lasts for the first few days to a few weeks following the stroke. During this stage, stroke patients generally are hospitalized and receive medical treatment to stabilize their condition. Caregivers play a critical role in this stage by ensuring the patient receives the appropriate medical care and support.

Subacute Stage

The subacute stage of stroke recovery usually begins once the patient is stable and discharged from the hospital. This stage can last from a few weeks to several months and is typically characterized by intensive therapy and rehabilitation. During this stage, stroke patients work with physical, occupational, and speech therapists to regain lost abilities and improve their overall function.

Chronic Stage

The chronic stage of stroke recovery begins once the patient has reached a plateau in their recovery and is no longer making significant progress. This stage can last indefinitely and requires ongoing management and support. Caregivers play a critical role in this stage by providing ongoing emotional support, helping with daily tasks, and ensuring that the patient's medical needs are met.

THE IMPORTANCE OF REHABILITATION

__My Story__ - Thank God I have always done some working out—weight training, yoga, ti chi, running, biking, all of it. I knew how to work out but also used to using a trainer. This is what rehabilitation is. It is not so much about what you do when you are with them but what you do when you are not. How much will you do to work through the pain on your own? How much will you research and work on to improve your situation? I ordered this stationary bike to start riding one week out of the hospital. You must be active, even if it hurts, and yes, it will hurt.

- Marc Parham

The importance of rehabilitation cannot be overstated regarding stroke recovery. Stroke patients who undergo rehabilitation are likely to experience better outcomes than those who do not. Rehabilitation can help stroke patients regain mobility, improve cognitive function, manage emotional distress, and overcome fatigue and weakness.

For men who have suffered a stroke, rehabilitation is crucial. Men are at a higher risk of stroke than women and often experience different symptoms. Men may also face unique challenges during recovery, such as mobility issues, cognitive impairments, and occupational limitations.

Rehabilitation can help men with mobility issues regain their ability to walk, climb stairs, and perform other activities of daily living. Physical therapy can help improve strength, balance, and coordination. Occupational therapy can help men learn adaptive techniques and tools to help them perform tasks they may have difficulty with.

Cognitive impairments can be a significant challenge for stroke patients, and men are no exception. Rehabilitation can help improve memory, attention, and other cognitive functions. Speech therapy can help men who have difficulty communicating.

Emotional distress is a common problem for stroke patients and can be particularly challenging for men. Men may be less likely to seek help for emotional issues, making recovery more difficult. Rehabilitation can help men manage feelings of depression, anxiety, and anger.

Fatigue and weakness are also common problems for stroke patients, and they can be particularly challenging for men with occupational limitations. Rehabilitation can help men improve endurance and energy levels, allowing them to participate more fully in work and other activities.

In conclusion, rehabilitation is an essential part of stroke recovery for men. It can help improve mobility, cognitive function, emotional well-being, and overall quality of life. Stroke patients and their caregivers should work closely with their healthcare providers to develop a rehabilitation plan that meets their unique needs and goals. With dedication and perseverance, stroke patients can thrive after a stroke.

Strategies for Setting Recovery Goals

My Story *- Setting goals will be difficult because you don't always know what you can do from one day to the next. Make sure to allow yourself the flexibility to modify your goals so you will not get frustrated. Some days, my goal was to walk on a treadmill for thirty minutes and then change to ten minutes because my endurance was not there. Listen to your body.*

- Marc Parham

Setting realistic recovery goals is crucial for stroke patients who want to thrive after a stroke. Stroke patients and their caregivers must understand that recovery is a journey that takes time and effort to achieve the desired outcome. Therefore, it is essential to set achievable goals that will motivate the patient to keep pushing forward.

The following strategies can help you and your caregivers set practical recovery goals:

You must consult with a healthcare professional

Consulting with a healthcare professional is vital in setting recovery goals. Not Dr. Google or Professor YouTube. This is because a healthcare professional will have a better understanding of your condition and can provide valuable advice on the type of goals that are realistic and achievable. Healthcare professionals can also help patients and their caregivers develop plans to achieve the set goals.

Focus on your strengths

It is essential to focus on your strengths when setting recovery goals. This will help you to stay motivated and build confidence in your abilities. For example, if you have good upper body strength, a goal could be to improve your ability to perform daily activities requiring the upper body.

Break down goals into smaller achievable tasks

Breaking down recovery goals into smaller achievable tasks can help you to stay motivated and focused. For example, if your goal is to walk independently, the first task could be to stand up without assistance, then take a few steps with assistance, and gradually increase the distance and time spent walking.

Set a timeline for achieving goals

Setting a timeline for achieving recovery goals can help you to stay focused and motivated. This timeline can change. Don't hold yourself to it. This is just a goal. A timeline can also help you and your caregiver to track progress and adjust the plan accordingly. It is important to be realistic when setting a timeline to avoid disappointment and frustration.

Celebrate milestones

Celebrating milestones is vital in keeping motivated. Celebrating small successes can help you to see progress and build confidence, which will help you to achieve bigger goals.

Celebrations can be as simple as praising or treating yourself to your favorite meal.

In conclusion, setting practical recovery goals is important in stroke recovery. You and your caregivers should consult with healthcare professionals, focus on your strengths, break down goals into smaller achievable tasks, set a timeline for achieving goals, and celebrate milestones. With the right mindset and strategies, you can thrive after a stroke.

How to stay motivated during recovery

My Story - *This is critical. You will have to find something that will keep you motivated. For me, it was a few things. Small things at first, like just picking up my guitar. It does not have to be big, but there has to be something to work towards. You are starting a new way of life.*

- Marc Parham

Recovering from a stroke can be a long and challenging journey, but it is important to stay motivated throughout the process. Motivation can come in many forms, such as setting goals, seeking support from loved ones or healthcare professionals, and finding ways to stay positive.

Here are some tips on how to stay motivated during recovery:

Seek support

Yes, I said it. Recovery can be a lonely journey, but it doesn't have to be. Seeking support from loved ones or healthcare professionals can provide emotional support and help you stay motivated. Joining a support group can also be a great way to connect with others who are going through a similar experience. Many online groups will help you by sharing their experiences. Just don't read, share. Sharing will help you.

Find ways to stay positive

Staying positive can be difficult when facing the challenges of recovery, but it is important to find ways to remain optimistic. This could mean practicing gratitude, focusing on the things you can do rather than what you can't, or finding humor in difficult situations.Take care of yourself

Recovery can be physically and emotionally exhausting, so it is important to take care of yourself. This could mean getting enough rest, eating a healthy diet, and finding ways to manage stress.

Stay engaged in activities you enjoy

Losing the ability to do things you enjoy can be a difficult part of recovery, but finding ways to stay engaged in activities you love is essential. This could mean adapting activities to fit your current abilities or finding new hobbies that you can enjoy.

In conclusion, staying motivated during recovery is essential to achieving your goals and maintaining a positive outlook. You can stay motivated throughout your recovery journey by setting realistic goals, seeking support, celebrating small victories, staying positive, taking care of yourself, and staying engaged in activities you enjoy.

STROKE RECOVERY FOR MEN WITH MOBILITY ISSUES

__My Story__ - This was a hard one for me. I was Mr. Mobile. I ran, I rode bikes, I hiked, I moved. To not be able to do this? And when I did, there was sometimes considerable pain. It is much easier to stay in bed —also the vanity issues about using handicapped devices. I was once in a store waking with my can, and a young man said, "Excuse me, pops," to get around me. I wanted to chase him with my cane, but I was already moving as fast as I could..lol.

- Marc Parham

Mobility limitations are a common challenge for stroke patients, especially for men. The inability to move around as freely as before can be frustrating, depressing, and isolating. However, coping with mobility limitations and maintaining a fulfilling and independent life after stroke is possible with the right strategies and support.

A man has to know his limitations.

Here are some tips to help stroke patients and their caregivers deal with mobility limitations:

Accept your limitations

Feeling frustrated, angry, or sad about the loss of mobility is natural. However, dwelling on negative emotions won't help you cope. Instead, accept your limitations and focus on what you can do. Be patient and give yourself time to adjust to your new reality.

Seek physical therapy

Physical therapy can help you regain strength, balance, and coordination and improve your ability to walk, stand, and move around. Work with a qualified physical therapist who understands your specific needs and goals.

Use assistive devices

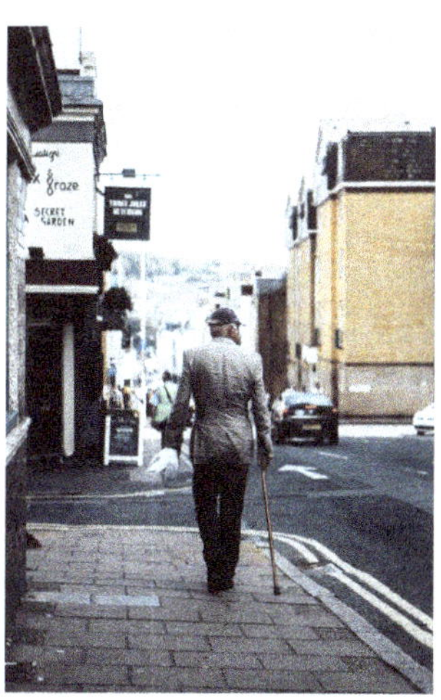

Many mobility aids can help you move around more efficiently and safely, such as canes, walkers, wheelchairs, and mobility scooters. Talk to your doctor or physical therapist about which device is best for you.

Modify your home

Making your home more accessible and safe can enhance mobility and independence. Consider installing grab bars, handrails, ramps, and stairlifts and removing obstacles and hazards.

Stay active

Even if you can't engage in vigorous exercise, it is important to stay active to maintain your physical and mental health. Try incorporating light exercises, such as stretching, seated, or gentle yoga, into your daily routine.

Stay connected

Mobility limitations can make you feel isolated and lonely. Stay connected with your friends, family, and community through social media, phone calls, or in-person visits. Join a support group or a recreational club that suits your interests and abilities.

Seek emotional support

Coping with mobility limitations can be emotionally draining. Seek emotional support from your loved ones, a therapist, or a support group. Talk about your feelings and concerns, and find ways to cope with stress and anxiety.

In conclusion, coping with mobility limitations after stroke requires a combination of acceptance, support, and practical strategies. With the right mindset and resources, stroke patients can maintain their independence, dignity, and quality of life.

Exercises for Improving Mobility

After a stroke, mobility is one of the most challenging issues for male stroke survivors. The ability to move freely and independently is essential for daily activities, and mobility is a key factor in overall quality of life.

Unfortunately, many stroke survivors experience significant mobility issues that can be frustrating and challenging.

Fortunately, some exercises can help improve mobility after a stroke. These exercises are designed to strengthen muscles and improve flexibility, balance, and coordination. With consistent practice, stroke survivors can regain mobility and independence.

Here are some exercises that can help improve mobility after a stroke:

Range of motion

The exercise involves moving each joint through its full range of motion. This can be done with simple movements like arm circles, leg swings, and shoulder shrugs.

Stretching

Stretching can help improve flexibility and range of motion. Stretching exercises should be done gently and gradually to avoid injury.

Strengthening exercises

These exercises focus on building strength in the muscles. They can be done with resistance bands, weights, or bodyweight exercises like squats, lunges, and push-ups.

Balance exercises

They are essential for mobility, and balance exercises can help improve stability and reduce the risk of falls. Balance exercises include standing on one leg, walking heel-to-toe, and standing on a wobbleboard.

Coordination exercises

These exercises focus on improving coordination and motor skills. They can include throwing and catching a ball, playing a musical instrument, or doing puzzles.

It's important to work with a physical therapist or healthcare professional to develop a safe and effective exercise program. They can help tailor exercises to a stroke survivor's specific needs and abilities.

In addition to exercise, other strategies can help improve mobility after a stroke. Using assistive devices like canes or walkers can help improve balance and stability. Modifying the home environment, such as installing grab bars or handrails, can also help reduce the risk of falls.

Mobility issues can be a significant challenge for stroke survivors, but with the right exercises and strategies, it's possible to regain independence and improve overall quality of life.

Tips for Adapting to Daily Life With Mobility Issues

My Story *- First, I had to accept the fact that I am handicapped. I may not be forever, but I will be for a long while. This was a hard pill to swallow. I had to get a handicap hangtag. Now I won't leave home without it. I still use my cane even though I am more stable. Especially when going to new places. It lets people know I move a little slowly and sometimes unstable. It also forces me to keep a certain cadence when walking. I carry a folding cane to pack it up when I don't need it.*

- Marc Parham

Mobility issues can be one of the most challenging aspects of stroke recovery for men. In addition to physical impairments, mobility issues can impact one's emotional and occupational well-being. However, with the right strategies, it is possible to adapt to daily life with mobility issues and maintain a fulfilling and independent lifestyle.

Here are some tips for stroke patients and caregivers to help adapt to daily life with mobility issues:

Please seek Professional Help

It is essential to consult with a healthcare professional to assess your mobility issues and develop a personalized rehabilitation plan. A physical or occupational therapist can help you identify your strengths and limitations and provide specialized exercises and techniques to improve your mobility.

Practice Safe Transfers

Transferring from one surface to another, such as from a bed to a wheelchair, can be challenging with mobility issues. It is essential to practice safe transfer techniques to prevent falls and injuries. A physical therapist can teach you proper transfer techniques that will help you maintain your independence.

Take Care of Your Emotional Well-being

Mobility issues can affect your emotional well-being. Seeking support from loved ones, friends, or a professional counselor is essential to help you cope with emotional distress. Joining a support group can also help connect with others who are going through similar experiences.

In conclusion, adapting to daily life with mobility issues after a stroke requires patience, perseverance, and a willingness to seek professional help. With the right strategies and support, it is possible to maintain independence and thrive in daily life.

Assistive Devices for Mobility

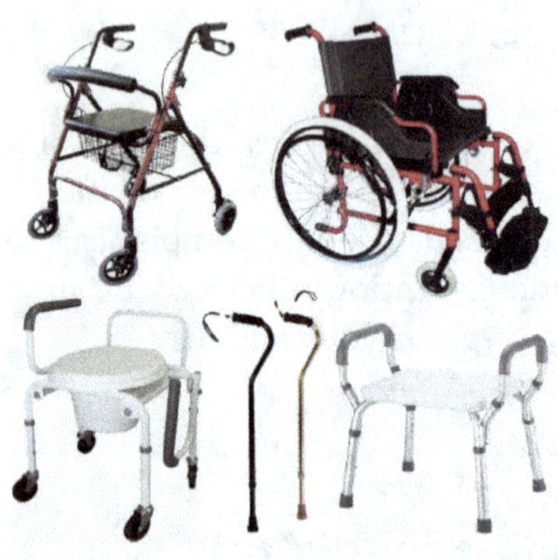

Assistive mobility devices can be a game changer in the stroke recovery process. They can allow stroke patients to move around their homes and communities more efficiently and independently. Various assistive devices are available, and it's important to find the ones that work best for each individual's needs.

One of the most common assistive devices for mobility is a wheelchair. Wheelchairs can be manual or electric, allowing stroke patients to move around their homes, communities, and workplaces. There are also specialized wheelchairs for specific needs, such as sports or showering.

Another type of assistive device is a walker or cane. These devices can provide support and stability for stroke patients with difficulty with balance and walking. They can also help to prevent falls and injuries.

A lift or transfer device may be necessary for stroke patients with more severe mobility issues. These devices can help to move stroke patients from their beds to a wheelchair or other location. They can also assist with activities of daily living, such as bathing and dressing.

In addition to these devices, there are also a variety of accessories that can help to make mobility more accessible and safer. For example, grab bars can be installed in bathrooms and other areas to provide support and stability. Non-slip mats can prevent falls, and ramps can be installed to make entrances and exits more accessible.

Working with healthcare providers and rehabilitation specialists is important to determine which assistive devices are appropriate for each individual's needs. They can guide how to use the devices and ensure they are used safely and correctly.

Assistive mobility devices can significantly improve stroke patients and their caregivers' quality of life. They can provide greater independence and make daily activities more accessible and manageable. With suitable devices and support, stroke patients can continue to thrive after their stroke.

STROKE RECOVERY FOR MEN WITH COGNITIVE IMPAIRMENTS

Understanding cognitive impairments after a stroke is crucial for stroke patients and their caregivers. Cognitive impairments refer to changes in how a person thinks, remembers, and solves problems. These changes may range from mild to severe, depending on the extent of the damage to the brain.

Stroke patients may experience cognitive impairments, impacting their daily life and ability to function independently. These impairments can manifest in different ways, including difficulty with memory, attention, and concentration and problems with language, perception, and reasoning.

The severity of cognitive impairments can vary depending on the location and extent of the stroke. For example, a stroke in the brain's left hemisphere may affect language skills, while a stroke in the right hemisphere may affect spatial awareness and perception.

Stroke patients must work with a healthcare provider to identify and manage cognitive impairments. This may include cognitive rehabilitation, a structured program that helps individuals improve their cognitive function. Cognitive rehabilitation may consist of activities such as memory exercises, problem-solving tasks, and language therapy.

Stroke patients may also benefit from making lifestyle changes to support cognitive health. This may include regular exercise, a healthy diet, and staying mentally active through reading, puzzles, or socializing with friends and family.

Caregivers play a crucial role in supporting stroke patients with cognitive impairments. They can help by providing a structured routine, simplifying tasks, and supporting and encouraging. Caregivers can also help stroke patients stay organized by creating lists and reminders and assisting with appointments and medications.

In conclusion, understanding cognitive impairments after a stroke is essential for stroke patients and their caregivers. Working with healthcare providers to identify and manage impairments, make lifestyle changes to support cognitive health, and provide support and encouragement to stroke patients is important. By working together, stroke patients and their caregivers can thrive after a stroke despite the challenges of cognitive impairments.

Strategies for Improving Memory, Attention, and Concentration

One of stroke patients' most common challenges is memory, attention, and concentration deficits. These defects can significantly affect an individual's ability to carry out daily activities, work, and engage in social activities. However, several strategies can help improve memory, attention, and concentration following a stroke.

Repetition

One of the most effective strategies for improving memory is repetition. This technique involves repeating information multiple times, either verbally or in writing. For example, if you need to remember someone's name, repeat it several times in your head or out loud. If you need to remember a list of items, write them down and read them repeatedly.

Chunking

Another strategy for improving memory is chunking. This technique involves breaking down complex information into smaller, more manageable pieces. For example, if you need to remember a phone number, break it into three or four-digit chunks.

Mindfulness

Mindfulness techniques such as meditation and deep breathing can help improve attention and concentration. These techniques help to calm the mind and reduce distractions, allowing you to focus better.

Physical exercise

Physical exercise is essential for overall health and well-being but can also help improve memory and concentration. Exercise increases blood flow to the brain, which can improve cognitive function.

Use of memory aids

Memory aids such as calendars, notes, and reminders can be helpful for individuals with memory deficits. These aids can help you remember important tasks, appointments, and events.

Social support

Social support from family, friends, and support groups can benefit stroke patients. Social interaction can help improve cognitive function and reduce emotional distress.

Occupational therapy

Occupational therapy can help stroke patients improve their memory, attention, and concentration skills. An occupational therapist can work with you to develop strategies to improve cognitive function and help you perform daily tasks more efficiently.

In conclusion, improving memory, attention, and concentration following a stroke requires a combination of strategies. Repetition, chunking, mindfulness, physical exercise, memory aids, social support, and occupational therapy can all be helpful for stroke patients. By implementing these strategies, stroke patients can improve their cognitive function and overall quality of life.

Coping With Communication Difficulties

Stroke patients often experience communication difficulties, which can be frustrating and isolating. If your loved one is struggling with aphasia or difficulty speaking, it can be challenging to know how to communicate with them. However, there are some simple strategies that you can use to help improve communication and help your loved one feel more connected and supported.

First, it is important to be patient and understanding. It can be frustrating for the patient and caregiver when communication is difficult, but it is important to remain calm and supportive. Try not to interrupt or finish their sentences, as this can be disempowering and make them feel as though they are not being heard.

Secondly, it is important to use non-verbal communication to help support your loved one. This can include using gestures, facial expressions, and body language to help convey meaning. For example, if your loved one struggles to find the right word, you can use a gesture or facial expression to help them understand what you are trying to say.

Thirdly, it can be helpful to use visual aids to support communication. This can include using pictures, diagrams, or written words to help your loved one understand what you are trying to say. This can be particularly helpful for stroke patients with cognitive impairments or memory problems.

Fourthly, using clear and straightforward language when communicating with stroke patients is essential. Avoid using complex or abstract language, which can be difficult for stroke patients to understand. Instead, use simple sentences and concrete language to help convey meaning.

Finally, seeking support from others who have experienced similar communication difficulties can be helpful. This can include joining a support group for stroke patients and caregivers or seeking advice from a speech therapist or other healthcare professional.

Communication difficulties can be a significant challenge for stroke patients and their caregivers. However, with patience, understanding, and the right strategies, it is possible to improve communication and help your loved one feel more connected and supported.

STROKE RECOVERY FROM MEN WITH EMOTIONAL DISTRESS

***My Story** - All I can say is WOW! My emotions are all over the place. Sometimes, I can't even talk without tearing up. One night, I watched Sheriff Taylor be upset with Opie about him not telling on his friends accused of burning down a barn. Tears just started rolling down my face. I can not control my emotions, so now I embrace them. I am breaking the Bro Code rules all over the place.*

- Marc Parham

The emotional impact of stroke on men can be devastating and often goes unnoticed. While

physical symptoms are commonly discussed, the emotional toll of stroke can be just as significant. Men who have suffered a stroke may experience a range of emotions, including frustration, anger, sadness, and anxiety.

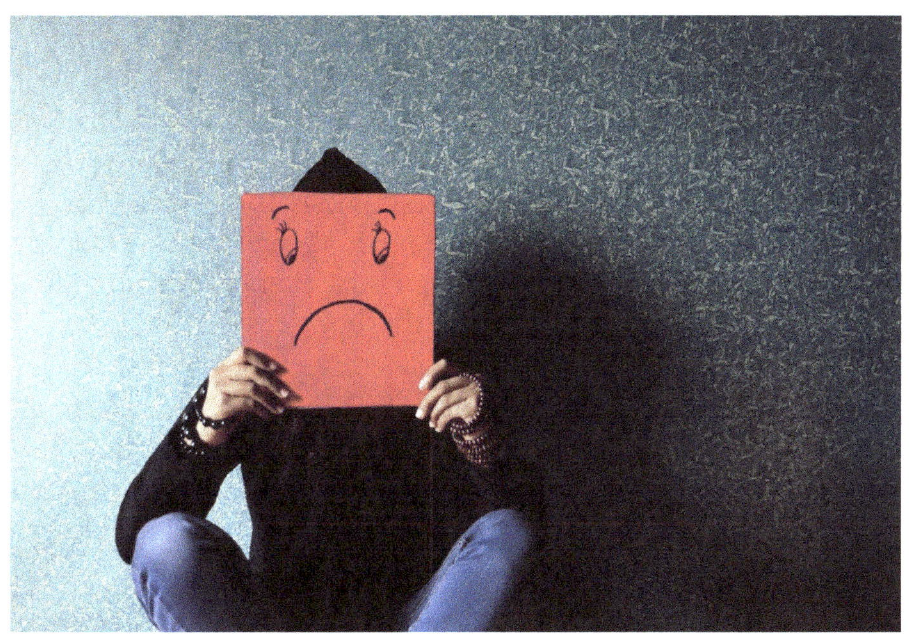

One of the most common emotional reactions to stroke is depression. This can be caused by a variety of factors, including changes in brain chemistry, loss of independence, and the stress of dealing with a life-altering event. Men may also feel a sense of grief or loss for their lives before the stroke, which can be challenging to come to terms with.

Another emotional issue that men may face after a stroke is anxiety. This can be caused by a fear of having another stroke, worries about their ability to care for themselves, and uncertainty about the future. Men may also experience social anxiety if they feel self-conscious about their physical limitations or cognitive impairments.

Men need to seek support and treatment for their emotional distress. This may include counseling, medications, or support groups. Caregivers can also play a critical role in helping men cope with their emotions by providing a listening ear, offering encouragement, and helping them stay engaged in activities that bring them joy.

Fatigue and weakness can also contribute to emotional distress in men who have suffered a stroke. These physical symptoms can make it difficult to participate in activities they enjoy, leading to feelings of isolation and depression. Caregivers can help by encouraging men to participate in physical therapy and providing support and encouragement along the way.

Occupational limitations can also significantly impact a man's emotional well-being. Losing the ability to work can be a blow to a man's sense of identity and purpose. Caregivers can help men find new hobbies or activities that bring them a sense of fulfillment and purpose.

In conclusion, the emotional impact of stroke on men is significant and should not be overlooked. Seeking support and treatment for emotional distress can be as important as physical rehabilitation. Caregivers can play a critical role in helping men cope with their emotions and find meaning and purpose in their lives after a stroke.

Strategies for Managing Depression and Anxiety

Depression and anxiety are common after-effects of a stroke and can significantly impact stroke patients and their caregivers' quality of life. However, stroke patients and caregivers can use several strategies to manage depression and anxiety and improve overall mental health.

Seek professional help

The first step in managing depression and anxiety is to seek professional help. This may involve talking to a therapist, counselor, or psychiatrist who can provide support and guidance on coping strategies and medication options.

Practice relaxation techniques

Deep breathing, meditation, and yoga can help reduce stress and anxiety. These techniques can be practiced at home or in a group setting, such as a yoga or meditation class.

Stay social

Social isolation can exacerbate symptoms of depression and anxiety. Staying connected with friends and family, joining support groups, or volunteering can help reduce feelings of loneliness and improve overall mood.

Set achievable goals

Setting big and small goals can help provide a sense of purpose and accomplishment. Setting realistic and achievable goals is important, as failure to meet them can lead to frustration and self-doubt.

Stay engaged in activities

Engaging in enjoyable activities, such as hobbies or interests, can help provide a sense of purpose and enjoyment. It's important to continue engaging in activities that were enjoyed before the stroke, as well as exploring new interests.

Follow a healthy diet

A healthy diet can help improve overall physical and mental health. Eating a well-balanced diet that includes plenty of fruits, vegetables, whole grains, and lean protein can provide the necessary nutrients to support mental health.

In conclusion, managing depression and anxiety after a stroke is an ongoing process that requires effort and commitment. Stroke patients and caregivers can improve overall mental health and well-being by seeking professional help, practicing relaxation techniques, staying social, setting achievable goals, staying engaged in activities, and following a healthy diet.

COPING WITH CHANGES IN RELATIONSHIPS AND INTIMACY

My Story *- With all these emotions running around, I have been breaking the Bro Code all over the place. I can't help but express my emotions now to anyone who listens. I am also not the man I used to be. This and other changes have made me hesitate to involve myself with new people. I never know how I will feel one day to the next, which is unfair to my friends. I also realize that when people ask how I am doing with that little tilt of the head, I don't have to tell them everything because whatever I am feeling may change in the next thirty minutes. I also provide full disclosure to prepare people for what may happen.*

- Marc Parham

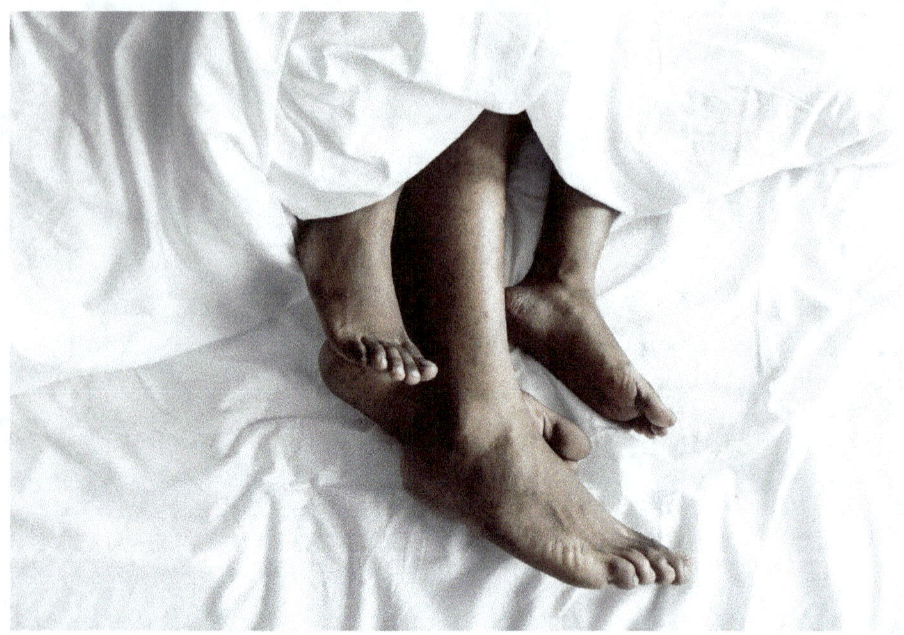

Stroke can bring about significant changes in an individual's relationships and intimacy. It can be challenging for stroke survivors and their caregivers to navigate these changes. However, it is essential to understand that these changes are common and can be addressed to ensure a fulfilling life after a stroke.

One of the most common changes experienced by stroke survivors is a shift in the relationship dynamic with their partner or spouse. It is not uncommon for the caregiver to take on a more significant role in the relationship, leading to a change in the dynamics that can be difficult to navigate. It is essential to have open and honest communication with your partner or spouse about these changes and how you can work together to maintain a healthy relationship.

Another issue that can arise after a stroke is changes in intimacy. This can be a complex topic to discuss, but it is crucial to address to maintain a healthy relationship. Stroke survivors may experience physical changes that affect their ability to engage in sexual activity. It is essential to have open communication with your partner or spouse about these changes. It may also be helpful to speak with a healthcare professional about potential solutions or adaptations that can be made to maintain intimacy.

Stroke recovery can also bring about emotional distress, leading to relationship changes. It is essential to seek support from a therapist or counselor to address and work through these emotional changes. It is also crucial to communicate with your partner or spouse about your emotional needs and how they can support you during this time.

Adapting to the home environment may be necessary for stroke survivors with mobility issues to ensure safe and comfortable intimacy. This may include the use of assistive devices or modifications to the physical environment. It is important to work with a healthcare professional or occupational therapist to identify potential adaptations that can be made.

Finally, stroke recovery can also bring about fatigue and weakness, leading to occupational limitations. Communicating with your partner or spouse about your limitations and working together to find solutions is essential. This may include delegating tasks or seeking outside assistance to ensure that both partners can maintain a healthy balance in the relationship.

In conclusion, coping with changes in relationships and intimacy after a stroke can be challenging, but it is essential to address these changes to maintain a fulfilling life. Open communication with your partner or spouse, seeking support from healthcare professionals, and adapting to the environment and daily routines can all help you navigate these changes. Remember, stroke recovery is a journey, and with patience, hard work, and support, a fulfilling life after a stroke is possible.

Building a Support Network

One of the most important things to remember when recovering from a stroke is that you don't

have to do it alone. Building a support network can make a huge difference in your recovery journey, especially for men facing unique challenges such as mobility issues, cognitive impairments, emotional distress, fatigue and weakness, and occupational limitations.

Your support network can consist of a variety of people, including family members, friends, healthcare professionals, and support groups. Each person in your network can offer different types of support and encouragement, which can help you overcome the various obstacles you may face during your recovery.

Family members can provide practical support, such as helping with household tasks or transportation to appointments. They can also offer emotional support by being there to listen, provide comfort, and encourage you to keep going. Friends can offer similar types of support and give a sense of normalcy and social interaction, which can be important for mental health.

Healthcare professionals such as doctors, nurses, and physical therapists can provide specialized support and guidance for your recovery. They can help you set achievable goals, monitor your progress, and offer treatment options to help you regain your strength and mobility.

Support groups can also be a valuable resource for stroke patients and caregivers. These groups can provide a sense of community and shared experiences, which can be comforting and empowering. They can also offer practical advice and tips for managing the challenges of stroke recovery.

No matter who is in your support network, it's essential to communicate your needs and goals with them. Be clear about what kind of support you need and how they can help you achieve your goals. Remember, stroke recovery is a journey, and having a solid support network can make all the difference in your success.

STROKE RECOVERY FOR MEN WITH FATIGUE AND WEAKNESS

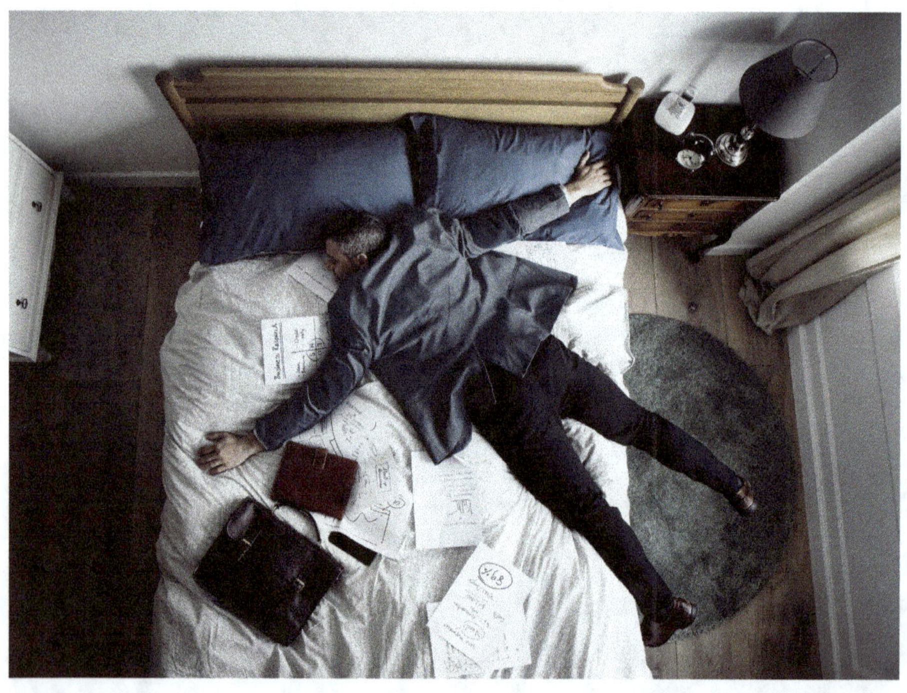

Fatigue and weakness are common symptoms that stroke survivors experience during their recovery. Understanding these symptoms and how they can affect your daily life is essential.

After a stroke, the brain undergoes changes that can cause fatigue and weakness. The brain controls the body's movements and energy levels, which can affect how the body functions when damaged. Fatigue and weakness can make it more difficult for stroke survivors to engage in routine activities.

Fatigue is a feeling of tiredness or exhaustion that can be physical or mental. Physical fatigue can make it hard to move or complete tasks, while mental fatigue can make it difficult to focus or remember things. Weakness is a lack of strength or power, making it hard to perform daily tasks.

Stroke survivors may experience fatigue and weakness in different ways. Some may feel tired after a short period of activity, while others may feel tired all the time.

Weakness may affect one side of the body more than the other, making it difficult to perform specific tasks.

Managing fatigue and weakness is essential to prevent them from affecting your daily life. Here are some tips to help you manage these symptoms:

Pace yourself

Break up activities into shorter sessions and take frequent breaks to avoid becoming too tired.

Get enough rest

Make sure you're getting enough sleep at night and rest during the day if needed.

Exercise

Regular exercise can help improve energy levels and reduce fatigue.

Eat a healthy diet

Eating a balanced diet can help provide your body with the nutrients it needs to function properly.

Manage stress

Stress can contribute to fatigue and weakness, so finding ways to manage it is important.

Talk to your healthcare provider

Your healthcare provider can help you manage your symptoms and recommend specific treatments if needed.

Fatigue and weakness can be challenging to manage, but you can improve your energy levels and quality of life with the right strategies. It's essential to be patient with yourself and take things one day at a time. You can overcome these symptoms and thrive after a stroke with time and effort.

Strategies for Increasing Energy Levels

One of the most common complaints among stroke patients is fatigue and weakness, which can significantly affect their ability to perform daily activities and engage in life. If you or your loved one struggles with fatigue and weakness after a stroke, several strategies can be implemented to increase energy levels and improve quality of life.

Stay hydrated

Dehydration can cause fatigue and weakness, so drinking enough water throughout the day is important. Aim for at least 8-10 glasses of water daily, and avoid caffeinated beverages that can dehydrate you.

Get enough sleep

Lack of sleep can worsen fatigue and weakness, so it's essential to get enough sleep each night. Aim for 7-8 hours of sleep and establish a regular sleep routine to help improve sleep quality.

By implementing these strategies, stroke patients and caregivers can work together to improve energy levels and overall quality of life. Remember that recovery after a stroke is a journey, and progress may be slow. With patience, perseverance, and support, it is possible to thrive after a stroke.

Exercises for Improving Strength and Endurance

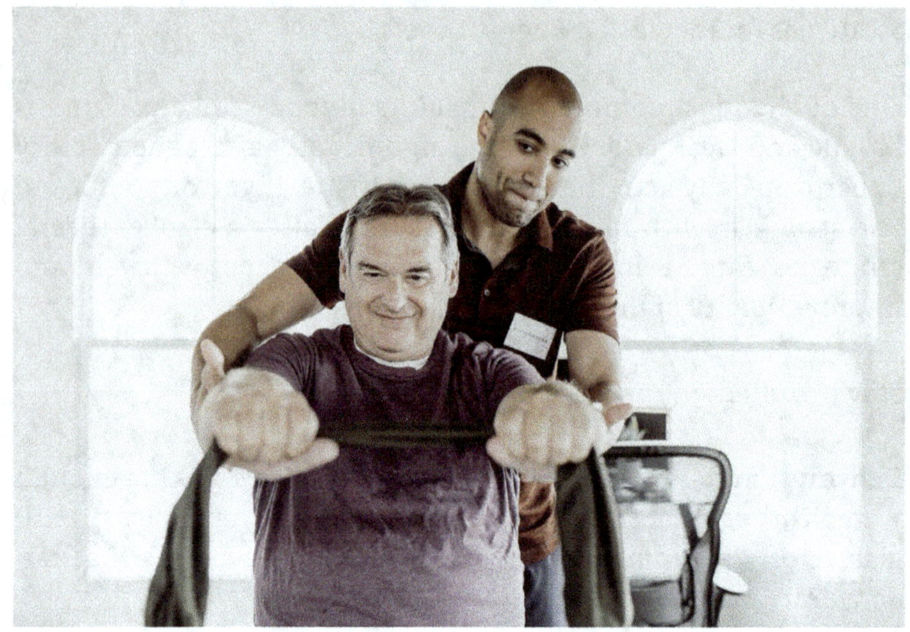

Improving strength and endurance is one of the most important aspects of stroke recovery. This can be a challenging process, but with the right exercises and guidance, it's possible to make significant improvements over time.

There are a variety of exercises that can help improve strength and endurance after a stroke. Here are a few examples:

Resistance training: This exercise involves using weights, resistance bands, or other tools to build strength in specific muscle groups. Resistance training can benefit stroke patients who have lost muscle mass or experienced weakness on one side of their body.

Aerobic exercise

Aerobic exercise, such as walking, cycling, or swimming, can be a great way to build endurance and improve cardiovascular health. It's important to start slowly and gradually increase the intensity and duration of your workouts over time.

Balance training

Many stroke patients experience balance issues, making it difficult to perform everyday activities. Balance training exercises, such as standing on one leg or practicing yoga poses, can help improve stability and reduce the risk of falls.

Functional training

Functional training involves performing exercises that mimic everyday movements, such as getting up from a chair or bending down to pick something up. By practicing these movements in a controlled environment, stroke patients can improve their strength and coordination.

Stretching

Stretching can help improve flexibility and range of motion, which can be especially important for stroke patients who experience muscle stiffness or spasticity.

Working with a physical therapist or other healthcare professional is important when starting an exercise program after a stroke. They can help you develop a personalized plan considering your needs and limitations.

In addition to these exercises, staying motivated and following a regular exercise routine is important. This can be challenging, especially for stroke patients who may experience fatigue or other limitations. However, by setting achievable goals and focusing on the benefits of exercise, it's possible to make progress and improve overall health and well-being.

STROKE RECOVERY FOR MEN WITH OCCUPATIONAL LIMITATIONS

Returning to work after a stroke can be one of the most challenging aspects of stroke recovery. It can be difficult to know where to start, what to expect, and how to navigate the challenges of returning to the workplace. However, with the right approach and support, it is possible to return to work after a stroke and thrive in your career.

Returning to work can be incredibly challenging for men who have experienced a stroke. Depending on the severity of the stroke and the resulting impairments, men may face mobility issues, cognitive impairments, emotional distress, fatigue and weakness, and occupational limitations. Understanding these challenges and developing a plan for addressing them is important.

One of the first steps in returning to work after a stroke is to assess your abilities and limitations. This may involve working with a physical or occupational therapist to develop a plan for building strength and improving mobility. It may also involve cognitive rehabilitation to address any memory or attention deficits.

In addition to physical and cognitive rehabilitation, emotional support is crucial in the return-to-work process. Men who have experienced a stroke may experience depression, anxiety, and other emotional challenges that can impact their ability to return to work. It is important to seek support from a mental health professional or support group to address these emotional challenges.

Fatigue and weakness are common challenges for men returning to work after a stroke. It is important to develop a plan for managing these symptoms, such as taking breaks throughout the day or adjusting work hours to accommodate for fatigue.

Occupational limitations, such as difficulty with fine motor skills or communication, may require accommodations in the workplace. This may involve working with an employer to modify job duties or providing assistive technology to improve communication.

Returning to work after a stroke can be a challenging and emotional process, but with the proper support and resources, it is possible to thrive in your career. By assessing your abilities and limitations, seeking emotional support, managing fatigue and weakness, and working with your employer to make accommodations, you can successfully return to work after a stroke.

Strategies for Finding New Career Opportunities

After a stroke, many men may feel like their career options are limited. However, with some

creativity and a willingness to explore new opportunities, it is possible to find fulfilling work. Here are some strategies for finding new career opportunities:

Consider your skills and interests: Start by taking an inventory of your skills and interests. What are you good at? What do you enjoy doing? This can help you identify potential career paths that align with your strengths and passions.

Network: Reach out to friends, family, and colleagues to let them know you are looking for new career opportunities. Attend industry events, job fairs, and networking events to expand your professional circle and learn about new job openings.

Volunteer

Volunteering can be a great way to gain new skills, build your professional network, and explore new career paths. Look for volunteer opportunities in your community that align with your interests and abilities.

Consider a career change

If your previous career is no longer feasible due to mobility, cognitive impairments, or other limitations, consider a career change. Look for growing industries with a high worker demand, such as healthcare, technology, or skilled trades.

Explore remote work options

If mobility or other limitations make commuting difficult to a traditional office job, consider remote work options. Many companies now offer remote work opportunities, allowing you to work from home or another location.

Seek support

Don't fear seeking permission from a career counselor, rehabilitation specialist, or other professional. They can help you identify new career opportunities and guide you through the job search process.

Finding a new career opportunity after a stroke may take time and patience. But with the right mindset and support, finding fulfilling work that aligns with your skills, interests, and limitations is possible.

CAREGIVING FOR MEN AFTER STROKE

My Story *- My abilities changed day to day. Things like walking and communicating were very up and down for me. I am sure it was challenging for my caregiver. Thinking I am getting better, and then one day, I am going backward. Some days, I was living in a fog. They call this "brain fog." After two years, I am still dealing with this. As a caregiver, you must remember that although we look okay, talk okay, and do other things okay, WE ARE NOT OK.*

- Marc Parham

A caregiver's role is critical in a stroke patient's recovery journey. As a caregiver, you provide the stroke patient with physical, emotional, and mental support. Your role is not limited to just assisting with daily activities but also being a constant source of motivation and encouragement during recovery.

For stroke patients with mobility issues, you may need to assist with physical therapy exercises, help with mobility aids, and ensure their safety during transfers. Communication is also essential, as you need to understand their limitations and how best to assist them.

For stroke patients with cognitive impairments, you may

need to assist with memory and cognitive exercises, help with communication, and ensure they follow their medication regimen. Patience is key in this role, as progress may be slow, and it may take time for the patient to regain their cognitive abilities.

Stroke patients with emotional distress may require extra emotional support, such as active listening and empathy. It is essential to encourage them to express their feelings and thoughts and provide a safe space to do so.

Stroke patients with fatigue and weakness may require assistance with daily activities, such as bathing and dressing. You may also need to encourage them to rest when necessary and maintain a healthy lifestyle to help improve their energy levels.

For stroke patients with occupational limitations, you may need to support finding alternative employment or modify their current job duties to accommodate their limitations.

Overall, the role of a caregiver is crucial in the recovery process. It requires patience, empathy, and understanding, but the rewards are immeasurable when you see the progress and improvements your loved one makes. Remember to take care of yourself as well, as the role of a caregiver can be physically and emotionally taxing. Seek support from family, friends, or support groups to help you maintain your own mental and physical well-being.

Coping with Caregiver Stress and Burnout

SELF CARE

Coping with caregiver stress and burnout is a common issue among stroke patients and their caregivers. Caring for a loved one who has experienced a stroke can be emotionally, physically, and mentally exhausting. Caregiver stress and burnout can occur when the caregiver is overwhelmed, overworked, and feels like they have no control over the situation.

To prevent caregiver stress and burnout, caregivers must take care of themselves. This can include taking breaks, getting enough sleep, exercising, and eating healthy. Caregivers should also seek support from family, friends, and support groups. Caregivers need to remember that they are not alone and that others are going through the same experience.

One of the biggest challenges for caregivers is balancing their own needs with the needs of the stroke patient. Caregivers need to set boundaries and communicate their needs to the stroke patient. This can include setting aside time for themselves and asking for help from others when needed.

Another way to cope with caregiver stress and burnout is to focus on the positive. Celebrate small victories and accomplishments, and take time to appreciate the good things in life. This can help to reduce stress and increase feelings of happiness and fulfillment.

Finally, caregivers need to seek professional help if they

are experiencing symptoms of depression or anxiety. Many resources are available, including therapists, support groups, and medication.

Coping with caregiver stress and burnout is challenging, but it is possible. By caring for yourself, setting boundaries, focusing on the positive, and seeking help, caregivers can overcome the challenges of caring for a loved one who has experienced a stroke.

Strategies for Providing Support and Encouragement

Recovering from a stroke can be a challenging experience, both for the patient and for their caregivers. However, providing support and encouragement is possible for a successful recovery with the right strategies.

One effective strategy is to establish clear goals and milestones for recovery. This can help to create an overall sense of progress and accomplishment, which can be a powerful motivator. Additionally, it is important to celebrate small successes along the way, such as regaining mobility or completing a challenging task. This can help to build confidence and keep the patient engaged and motivated.

Another critical strategy is to provide emotional support and encouragement. This can involve simply listening and offering words of encouragement, or it may include helping the patient find additional resources or support groups to provide additional emotional support. It is important to remember that recovery from a stroke can be long and challenging, and the patient may experience a wide range of emotions. By offering understanding and support, caregivers can help to provide a sense of stability and comfort during this difficult time.

In addition to emotional support, it is also important to provide practical assistance as needed. This may involve helping with daily tasks such as cooking, cleaning, transportation, medical appointments, or physical therapy sessions. By providing this practical support, caregivers can help reduce patient stress and fatigue, which in turn can help support their overall recovery.

Finally, it is essential to remember that recovery from a stroke is a unique and individual process, and what works for one patient may not work for another. By remaining flexible and open to new strategies and approaches, caregivers can help provide the customized support and encouragement each patient needs to thrive. With practical assistance, emotional support, and a focus on clear goals and milestones, caregivers can help their loved ones successfully navigate the challenges of stroke recovery and move toward a brighter future.

Building a Strong Caregiver-Patient Relationship

Building a strong caregiver-patient relationship is essential to the recovery of stroke patients. The bond between a caregiver and patient should be supportive, respectful, and built on trust. A strong relationship between a caregiver and a patient can help to reduce stress, anxiety, and depression and promote a positive outlook towards rehabilitation.

Here are some tips for building a strong caregiver-patient relationship:

Open Communication: Communication is the key to building a strong caregiver-patient relationship. It is essential to have open and honest communication to ensure that both the caregiver and patient understand each other's needs and expectations. Caregivers should listen to the patient's concerns, feelings, and needs and provide them with the support they need to recover.

Empathy: Empathy is the ability to understand and share the feelings of others. Caregivers should try to put themselves in the patient's shoes and understand what they are going through. This will help the caregiver to provide the support the patient needs, and the patient will feel understood and cared for.

Patience: Stroke patients may have physical, cognitive, or emotional challenges that can frustrate them and their caregivers. Caregivers need to be patient and allow them to work at their own pace. Encouragement and praise are essential to keep the patient motivated and help them overcome their challenges.

Respect: Respect is essential to building a strong caregiver-patient relationship. Caregivers should treat patients with dignity and respect and avoid being condescending or patronizing. Patients should be involved in decisions about their care, and their opinions and choices should be respected.

Building a strong caregiver-patient relationship is not always easy, but it is essential to the recovery of stroke patients. Caregivers need to be supportive, empathetic, patient, and respectful. Patients need to feel understood and cared for, and their needs and expectations should be met. With a strong caregiver-patient relationship, stroke patients can overcome their challenges and thrive after a stroke.

The Importance of Self-Care

The importance of self-care cannot be overemphasized when it comes to stroke recovery. Self-care refers to any activity that you engage in to maintain and improve your physical, mental, and emotional health. It involves taking care of yourself in ways that promote well-being and prevent illness and injury.

For stroke patients, self-care is essential to promote recovery and reduce the risk of future strokes. It is also crucial for caregivers to take care of themselves, as caregiving can be physically and emotionally draining. Here are some reasons why self-care is critical during stroke recovery:

Physical Health

Stroke patients often experience mobility issues, weakness, fatigue, and other physical challenges. Self-care activities such as regular exercise, healthy eating, and getting enough rest can help improve physical health and promote recovery.

Mental Health

Stroke patients may also experience cognitive impairments such as memory loss, difficulty with communication, and trouble processing information. Engaging in activities that stimulate the brain, such as reading, playing games, and socializing, can help improve cognitive function and mental health.

Emotional Health

Stroke recovery can be emotionally challenging, and many patients experience depression, anxiety, and other mood disorders. Engaging in activities that promote relaxation and stress reduction, such as meditation, yoga, and deep breathing exercises, can help improve emotional well-being.

Occupational Limitations: Stroke patients may also experience limitations in their ability to perform everyday tasks such as cooking, cleaning, and personal care. Engaging in activities that promote independence and self-sufficiency, such as occupational therapy and assistive technology, can help improve quality of life.

In conclusion, self-care is essential for stroke patients and caregivers alike. It is critical to prioritize self-care activities that promote physical, mental, and emotional well-being to promote recovery and prevent future strokes. Remember, taking care of yourself is not selfish; it is necessary for a successful recovery.

Encouragement for Continued Recovery

After a stroke, recovery can be a long and challenging journey. It is a time filled with uncertainty, fear, and frustration. However, it is important to remember that recovery is possible, and with the right mindset, tools, and support, you can make significant progress.

For stroke patients, the most important thing is to stay positive and motivated. It is natural to feel discouraged at times, but it is essential to keep pushing forward. You have already come a long way, and with perseverance and determination, you can continue to make progress.

For caregivers, your role is critical in providing the emotional and practical support needed for continued recovery. Your loved one may sometimes feel overwhelmed, frustrated, and even hopeless. It is important to be patient, compassionate, and understanding. Encourage and celebrate even the most minor achievements, and help them build a support system.

Stroke recovery for men with mobility issues can be particularly challenging. However, significant progress can be made with the right therapy and equipment. Physical therapy can help improve strength, balance, and coordination, while mobility aids such as walkers, canes, and wheelchairs can help make movement easier and safer.

Stroke recovery for men with cognitive impairments can be equally challenging. Memory loss, difficulty with communication, and problems with judgment and decision-making can make daily activities frustrating and overwhelming. However, cognitive therapy can help improve cognitive function, and assistive devices such as calendars, reminder apps, and communication aids can help make daily life easier.

Stroke recovery for men with emotional distress, such as depression, anxiety, and anger, can be particularly challenging. It is essential to address emotional issues as part of the recovery process. Counseling and support groups can help manage emotions and provide a safe space to express feelings.

Stroke recovery for men with fatigue and weakness can be frustrating. However, energy levels can be improved with proper exercise and rest. Occupational therapy can help identify energy-saving techniques and improve daily functioning.

Stroke recovery for men with occupational limitations can be challenging. However, with suitable accommodations, work can be possible. Vocational rehabilitation can help identify work options and provide workplace accommodations.

In conclusion, recovery after a stroke is possible with the right mindset, tools, and support. Stay positive, stay motivated, and never give up. With perseverance and determination, you can continue to make progress and thrive after a stroke.

Resources for Stroke Patients and Caregivers

Resources for stroke patients and caregivers are essential for the successful recovery and management of stroke-related issues. These resources can help stroke patients and caregivers navigate the complexities of stroke recovery, provide emotional support, and improve their quality of life. Here are some resources that stroke patients and caregivers can utilize:

Stroke Support Groups: Stroke support groups are an excellent resource for stroke patients and caregivers. These groups allow stroke survivors and caregivers to share their experiences, gain emotional support, and learn from others who have gone through similar situations. These groups can be found in hospitals, community centers, and online.

Stroke Rehabilitation Centers: Stroke rehabilitation centers offer a range of services to help stroke patients recover and manage their symptoms. These services include physical, occupational, speech, and counseling. Rehabilitation centers can be found in hospitals, clinics, and community centers.

Online Resources: Several online resources stroke patients and caregivers can use to access information and support. These resources include websites, forums, and social media groups dedicated to stroke recovery and caregiving.

Caregiver Support Services: Caregiver support services offer assistance and resources to caregivers caring for stroke patients. These services include respite care, support groups, counseling, and educational resources.

Stroke Associations: Stroke associations are non-profit organizations that provide resources, support, and advocacy for stroke patients and caregivers. These associations can help stroke patients and caregivers access information, find support groups, and connect with other stroke survivors.

Adaptive Equipment: Adaptive equipment can help stroke patients with mobility issues or cognitive impairments. These devices include mobility aids, communication devices, and assistive technology.

Stroke patients and caregivers need to utilize these resources to help them navigate the challenges of stroke recovery. Using these resources, stroke patients and caregivers can improve their quality of life and achieve successful recovery.

CONCLUSION

Simple Rules to Follow. Following are a few rules that I had to learn how to track and continue to follow to make the best of my recovery. I suggest you make rules for yourself that you will turn to when things get complicated. Believe me, they will get hard. There will also be amazing days ahead. I tell people that I feel like I have come out of this situation much smarter than I came in.

- ✓   **I know** more about myself physically, mentally, and emotionally.

- ✓   **I know** more about my health and how to maintain a healthy lifestyle.

- ✓   **I know** more about personal relationships and how they really work.

- ✓ **I know** more about my strengths and weaknesses and reach the goals that I have set for myself.

- ✓   **I know more about ME!**